5-Minute
FACELIFT

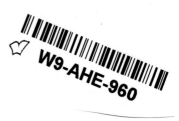

5-Minute
FACELIFT

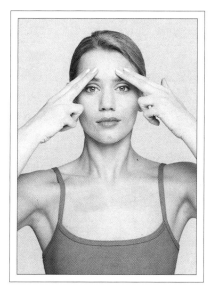

Robert Thé

Sterling Publishing Co., Inc.
New York

Photography: Antonio Traza

Models: Kitsa Pateras, Joanne Emma Ray, Dolores Serrallé, Mercedes Cabral-of-Smith, Sylver, Gemma Godas Villaverte, Steve Young

Make up: Sally Riceman

For Virgin Publishing: Carolyn Price

Design: Paul Kime

Library of Congress Cataloging-in-Publication Data Available

10 9 8 7 6 5 4 3 2 1

Published in 1997 by
Sterling Publishing Company, Inc
386 Park Avenue South,
New York, N.Y. 10016

Originally published in Great Britain in 1997 under the title *Five Minute Facelift* by Virgin Books
Text ©1995 by Robert Thé
Virgin Publishing Ltd

Distributed in Canada by
Sterling Publishing
c/o Canadian Manda Group,
One Atlantic Avenue, Suite 105
Toronto, Ontario, Canada M6K 3E7

Printed and bound in Italy

Sterling ISBN 0-8069-0451-8

This book is dedicated to Smita Joshi whose spirit is a testimony to youthfulness.

A book is the product of many people's ideas and efforts, and this one is no exception. I would like to acknowledge and thank the following for all their time, ideas and creative input:

Carmel Dungan
Julia Ahmad Jamal
Smita Joshi
Paul Kime
Kundan & Narendra Mehta
Kitsa Pateras
Carolyn Price
Sally Riceman
Dolores Serrallé
Dorita Sheriff
Mercedes Cabral-of-Smith
Martin Stollery
Antonio Traza
Nadia Warner
Steve Young

Robert Thé
London, 1997

CONTENTS

INTRODUCTION

In the past if you wanted to take care of your face as you got older you were limited to two basic options. With option A you could spend lots of money on very expensive and highly dubious anti-ageing creams for which many extravagant claims were made but which unfortunately usually brought only cosmetic and temporary benefits.

Option B was more drastic: when you felt that things were getting out of hand, facially speaking, you could arrange to have a surgical facelift. By a nip here and a tuck here, magic could be created: worrisome lines, wrinkles and sagging cheeks vanished overnight. The catch with this outrageously expensive procedure was that it had to be repeated every few years, tucking a bit more here and a slightly more there. What had started out as a solution often ended up being a major problem in its own right, as successive operations rapidly diminished the credit balance and created a progressively more mask-like face, each one more rigid and unnatural than the last.

But now there is a third way, a way based on sensible, natural methods that aim to preserve your good features for as long as possible. This method is easy to learn and can be practised by anyone, anywhere and at any point in their life. It enables us to take positive steps through exercise, to discourage signs of ageing before they have an opportunity to develop in youthful skins, and, in skins where they have developed, to minimize their effects.

How to use this book

This book is divided into three parts.

In the first part we hear about 'Modern Day Skin Stories' and discover the secret world of our skin, what its structure is, what factors are instrumental in ageing it, what a good basic skincare programme consists of and how our thoughts affect the quality of our skin. In 'Your Best Asset' we learn about the structure of the face, discovering the individual major muscles, what they do, where they are as well as seeing how they work together as a team, helping us express ourselves.

The middle of the book focuses on three different facial programmes which are designed to ensure that as we get older our skin remains in optimum condition. In 'Basic Facial Fitness' we work systematically through each major muscle of the face so that the whole face becomes toned. This is followed by 'Turning Back the Clock', which includes exercises designed to troubleshoot a range of common problems that can be experienced as we get older. This section includes special techniques that work on releasing deep tension in the connective tissue, tension that is often responsible for hard-to-hide wrinkles and lines. In 'Facial Harmony' we include massage techniques – using both oil and oil-free moves – that can restore radiance to your face.

In the final part, 'Less is More', we look at how make up can be used in a subtle way to enhance your positive features and reveal your full potential.

To obtain the best results from this book –

- Read through 'Modern Day Skin Stories' first.
- Start the skincare programme recommended.
- Begin with the 'Basic Facial Fitness' programme.
- Read through each exercise before attempting it.
- Make sure you have short nails and clean hands before you touch your face.
- Apply a little moisturizer before you start.
- Use a mirror to see yourself as you do the exercises.
- Repeat each exercise several times until the individual muscle tires.
- Use your imagination as well to help bring about changes.
- Practise as often as possible.
- Be patient: changes will happen through time.

My personal recommendation is that you work through the book systematically, chapter by chapter. The exercises form part of a structured programme and will not make sense if you tackle them randomly. As you work through the book you should begin to notice small changes occurring, and the longer you continue the more pronounced these should become.

I hope that you will enjoy using this book for many years to come and that, as you begin to notice the benefits of this powerful program, you will get everyone around you involved and regularly practising the Five Minute Facelift. So dive in, enjoy and here's to your health!

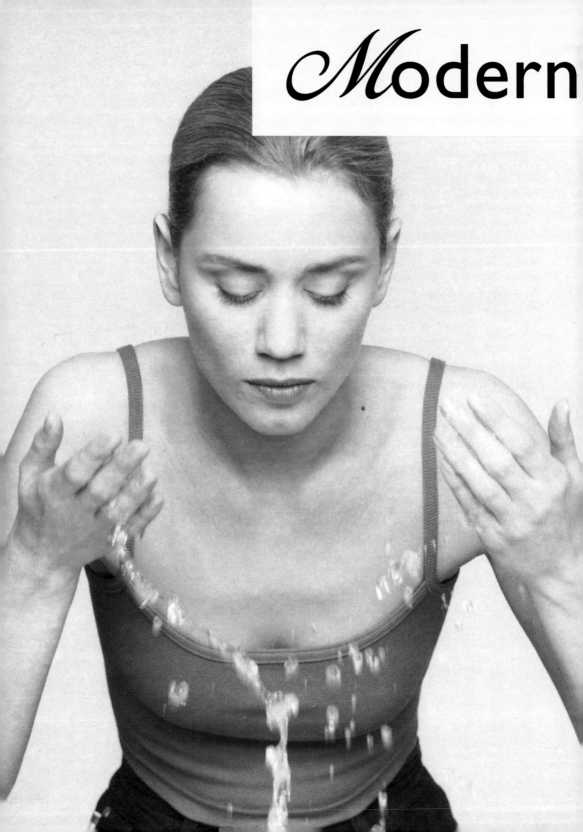

Modern

Day Skin Stories

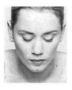

*I*magine for a moment that you really did wear your heart on your sleeve. It's a safe bet that you'd take good care of this precious, delicate organ and treat it with the respect it truly deserves.

But most people treat their skin, which is located on the outside of the body, as if it were unworthy of being cared for, paying it little if any attention. This is surprising because it is the largest of all the organs in the body, covering approximately two square meters (18 square feet) and weighing in at a hefty 3.2 kilos (7 pounds).

Your skin would be well within its rights to ask for compensation. It has a lot to contend with: regular exposure to the elements, filtering out harmful radiation and dealing with life's low life, such as dirt, grime and bacteria.

Despite everything the skin does for them, very few people take the time or effort to really understand it: how it ages, how to care for it and how best to listen to all the stories it has to tell. Understanding your skin is the first step in being able to care for it, of being able to lay strong foundations so that it remains healthy throughout your life. Practising preventative skin care on a daily basis, in conjunction with using the basic facial fitness programme and other exercises, will help you to maintain a healthy, glowing complexion and retain your good looks through the years.

No one could wish for a better bodyguard than the skin, which offers us head-to-toe protection, even when we sleep. And, like all the best bodyguards, the skin is not quite what it seems: outwardly supple and thin enough to allow complete freedom of movement, yet tough enough to offer a resilient waterproof barrier that stops life-essential water from getting out and undesirable things such as bacteria, infectious diseases and harmful ultraviolet radiation from getting in.

The skin is not just a simple surface covering the entire body: its thickness depends largely on where it is found, with the thickest skin occurring on the soles and palms and the thinnest around our eyelids. The skin is also a very busy place: in just one square centimetre there are approximately 3 million cells, 13 oil glands, 9 hairs, 100 sweat glands and 2.75 metres (3 yards) of nerves, 1 metre of blood vessels and thousands of sensory cells which allow minute differences of temperature, touch, pressure and pain to be instantly detected, providing accurate up-to-the-minute information about what is going on in the big wide world.

There's more to the skin than meets the eye. To begin with, what we normally think of as the skin is only the first or surface layer of several different layers. These first few layers form what is known as the epidermis, after that comes the dermis, then the subcutaneous layer containing fat cells that serve to protect the organs lying under it from damage.

The function of the epidermis is to offer a barrier, the first level of protection. The first layer, the stratum corneum, is made up of dead skin cells, which are continuously being shed. In fact, most household dust, when ana-lyzed, is found to be composed of these dead cells! The epidermis also contains specialized cells that create a pigment called melanin. The amount of melanin in our skin is what determines our skin colour. Exposure to ultraviolet light stimulates production of melanin which produces the effect of tanning, the body's protective response against ultraviolet radiation. In geographical areas where sunlight is intense, the indigenous populations have a lot of melanin in their skin, giving them a dark hue. Equally, people who live in temperate, less sunny zones tend to have less melanin present in their skin. However, to call the skin colour of such people 'white' is incorrect: it is often more of a pinkish hue, caused by the blood present in the dermis.

The dead cells at the surface of our skin are generated five layers below in the stratum basale, which is in charge of producing new skin cells. Some cells become specialized, like sweat or oil glands or hair follicles, while the remainder become general skin cells and set off on a four-week journey upwards through various levels until they reach the surface as dead skin cells.

Living in the city can sometimes cause the skin surface to become clogged with grease and dirt, and develop a dull, lifeless appearance. In addition to regular cleansing, exfoliation or dry skin brushing can help clear the skin of dead cells, stimulate blood and nutrient supply, clear toxins through improved lymphatic drainage and allow the skin to breathe freely. But the removal of dead skin cells has to be done in moderation: too zealous or frequent removal puts pressure on the basale layer and makes the skin sensitive and raw, and susceptible to ageing.

The dermis is often known as the true skin and is usually much thicker than the epidermis. Its main function is to provide support for the epidermis and various structures found within the dermis. It is mainly made up of connective tissue that binds together, supports, strengthens and gives general shape to our flesh. Contained within it are two protein-based fibres, collagen and elastin. These offer the skin the twin benefits of stretchability (the ability to put on weight or get pregnant without ripping or otherwise damaging the skin) and elasticity (the ability for the skin to return to its original shape after stretching).

Embedded within the matrix of the connective tissue are other specialized skin cells such as hair follicles and roots, touch and pressure sensitive nerve endings, veins, fat cells, arteries and various capillaries as well as sudiferous (sweat) and sebaceous (oil) glands.

There are approximately three to four million sudiferous glands in the body and these are mainly located in the subcutaneous layer. Their secretions are emptied via a duct that leads directly to a pore on the skin surface, and is a vital element in helping to regulate body temperature by providing a way of reducing it quickly.

Sebaceous glands are small sacs with a duct connected to hair follicles. They are found nearly everywhere on the surface of the body, particularly the face. These glands produce sebum, an oily lubricant that prevents the hair from becoming dry as well as creating a waterproof mantle for the skin which helps keep it soft and supple. The level of sebum production largely determines our skin type, whether it will be dry or oily.

The skin is remarkably resilient, able to repair itself rapidly, often leaving no apparent mark of any damage being done. But with all its strengths, the skin needs to be taken care of and respected. The attention and care we give it can directly improve the quality of our general health and the way we look. And so, far from being a luxury, the skin's complexity demands that it is looked after and cared for. By working to keep our skin in excellent condition, the collagen in the connective tissue can remain well-organized and supple as we get older instead of becoming rigid, brittle and knotted. This means we will develop fewer wrinkles and retain a handsome face for many years to come.

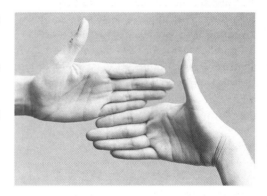

If your skin is oily, count yourself lucky. Not day-to-day lucky, but long-term lucky. Unlike dry skin, oily skin tends to take a lot longer to wrinkle and show signs of ageing. The same contrast can be found in people with olive or darker complexions who generally age at a slower rate than those with pale, light skin.

However, apart from our skin type, there are other biological factors involved in ageing which can be prepared for, thus affecting how quickly we age.

The first signs that we are getting older generally occur around the age of 25. Expression lines, caused by the constant wear and tear generated by using our facial muscles every day begin to appear, usually around the mouth and eyes. And there are also changes in the natural elasticity of our skin as this daily wear and tear begins to take its toll on the elastin in the skin, causing it to break down. When combined with a general loss of facial muscle tone, the skin can become a little looser than previously. However, this process can be slowed down considerably by regularly practising good skincare and following a basic facial fitness programme.

The thirties and forties often bring a maturity to the face as life experiences and lifestyle choices begin to etch themselves into our features. Expression lines deepen, more and more wrinkles appear and the skin can begin to show the cumulative effects of gravity, leading to local sagging and bags under the eyes.

The sudden hormonal upheaval of the menopause not only has a dramatic effect on the body, it can also trigger major changes within the face as well: the skin can become dryer or change its type completely; reduced circulation can lead to a paler complexion; collagen and fat cells in the face become reduced in size and number which, when combined with a general thinning of the skin, can cause the face to start to lose its natural plumpness, becoming slightly gaunt in appearance and triggering other signs of ageing to slowly develop: jowls, downturned mouths and turkey necks. Putting on a little extra as you get older is not such a bad idea, especially as it can help to counter the problem of natural shrinkage and collagen loss, plumping and filling out the skin. In addition, practising the basic facial fitness programme regularly and targeting specific problems using the trouble-shooting techniques shown in pages 46-60 will help to slow the effects of this change on the face.

Our lifestyle and environment also play a large part in determining how we age and how our skin responds. The principal environmental factor is the level of exposure to the sun's rays we experience throughout our lives. While limited protected exposure can be healthy, unprotected exposure and sunburn is most definitely not. Unprotected exposure to the sun can lead to the skin becoming dehydrated, the collagen within the connective tissues breaking down rapidly, and the appearance of wrinkles. So if you want to save your skin when out in the sun, always follow the Australian Slip, Slop, Slap rule: slip on a shirt or blouse, slap on a hat, and slop on the sun blocker. The higher the protection factor on the blocker, the better – even on cold, cloudy days.

In addition to the sun, the air that surrounds us and the air that we breathe plays an important role in the health of our skin.

Scientific findings show that smoking, whether active or passive, can age you just as rapidly as exposure to the sun, so is best avoided. Equally undesirable is the air conditioning and central heating found in most modern offices and homes. Although originally designed to make our immediate environment more pleasant, they tend to wreck havoc with our skin by drying it out. If your workplace or home has air-conditioning or central heating, make sure you regularly moisturize your skin and get plenty of fresh air, to counterbalance the effect of an indoor climate.

Eating poor quality, highly processed food such as convenience meals or fast food can also have a marked effect on our skin, because these often lack fibre and contain high levels of saturated fats, questionable additives and refined sugar, which the body regards as highly toxic, rejecting it often in the form of facial spots. Unsurprisingly, this type of diet often leaves your skin and face looking dull and starved of life. If your aim is to look as vibrant and healthy as possible, then include in your daily diet as much natural, fresh, unrefined food as possible. This will give your body the vitamins, nutrients and fibre it needs to keep you looking at your best.

Given that we are made up of 70 per cent water, what we drink has a significant effect on the quality of our skin and how we age. Drinks like tea and coffee, which contain toxins, are better avoided, as is alcohol, which has a negative physical effect on our body, causing it to rapidly dehydrate. The human body appreciates the intake of fresh water (between 1.5 and 2 litres/2-3 pints) every day to help the kidneys flush toxins from the system. This will leave the skin clearer and no tell-tale dark bags under the eyes to show that the kidneys are having a hard time dealing with all the toxins in your system. A regular monthly one-or two-day detox and system cleanse using just natural fruit juices or water also works wonders for your skin. Ask your doctor on how best to start.

The skin is a very accurate barometer of how stressed we are and will rapidly show when you are under too much pressure. If this pressure is sustained at too high a level for too long then, as many high-fliers often find to their cost, it can trigger rapid ageing, especially in the face. The antidote to stress is to make sure you manage it on a regular and continual basis, learning to relax fully. If you don't, then your skin is likely to suffer and wrinkles will settle in as long-term tenants. Getting regular, quality sleep should be a major part of your relaxation programme, because it helps the body to rest, recover and heal itself. Not for nothing do models hit the pillows early every evening: they know that it's the best way to make sure their skin is always in top form.

An optimum lifestyle doesn't happen overnight, it takes small constant changes and improvements: a nudge here and a nudge there to go in the right direction, and a sense of flexibility to forgive yourself for drifting off course occasionally. But, by making lifestyle choices that are kind to your skin, you will be doing yourself a big favour, long-term. And as the seasons change, your face will begin to show the benefits of all the positive choices you have made through the years.

𝒜 regularly followed skincare routine used in conjunction with the basic facial fitness programme is essential if you want your skin to look fresh and vibrant now and in the future. A basic programme involves: cleansing to remove excess make-up, dirt and grime, toning to remove the cleanser, and moisturizing which keeps the skin smooth and supple, discouraging wrinkles; exfoliation removes dead skin cells from the surface, and a mask detoxes and purifies the skin. Regular cleansing involves steps 1–4, which should be done twice a day. Exfoliate and use a mask twice a week, following the steps in this order: 1, 2, 5, 6, 3 and 4.

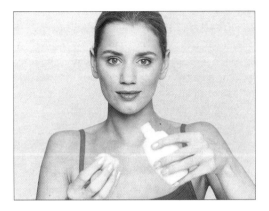

| Cleanse: Remove make-up and dirt build-up with cleanser.

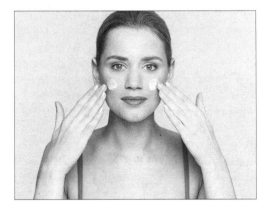

4 Moisturize: Use an appropriate mositurizer to hydrate the skin and help seal moisture in.

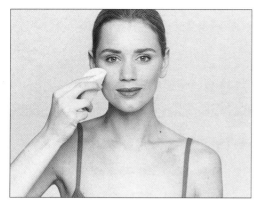

2 Wipe: Using a warm cloth, wipe face.

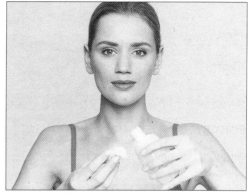

3 Tone: Using a toner on cotton balls, gently go over face, avoiding the eye area.

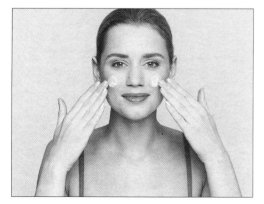

5 Exfoliate: Choose an exfoliant that suits you, and avoid rubbing harshly on cheeks and eye area. Remove with warm water.

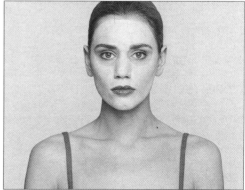

6 Mask: Avoiding the eye area, apply a mask to dry skin. After the impurities have been drawn, remove thoroughly with warm water, tone and moisturize as usual.

THINKING BEAUTY

 *T*rue beauty is not just about how you look on the outside, but how you feel on the inside. What's going on the inside is easy to spot, especially when we're upset or worried. The ability to take control of any thoughts that may push us off balance or which are less than positive is very important. Learning to release internal negativity can help us to release physical tension, especially within our face, and is the first step in learning how to allow our inner beauty to radiate outwards. So, let go of the strains of the day and think only beautiful thoughts as you try the following exercises.

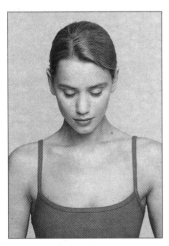 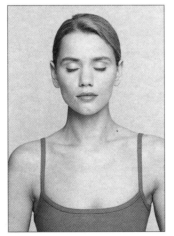 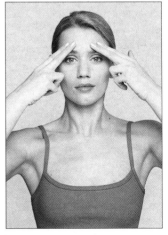

1 Sit with your head upright and very slowly lower your head.

2 Raise your head back up at the same speed, breathing slowly. Stop when your head is level again.

3 Finally, press two fingers just above each browbone and hold for a few minutes. These are excellent points to calm and centre you.

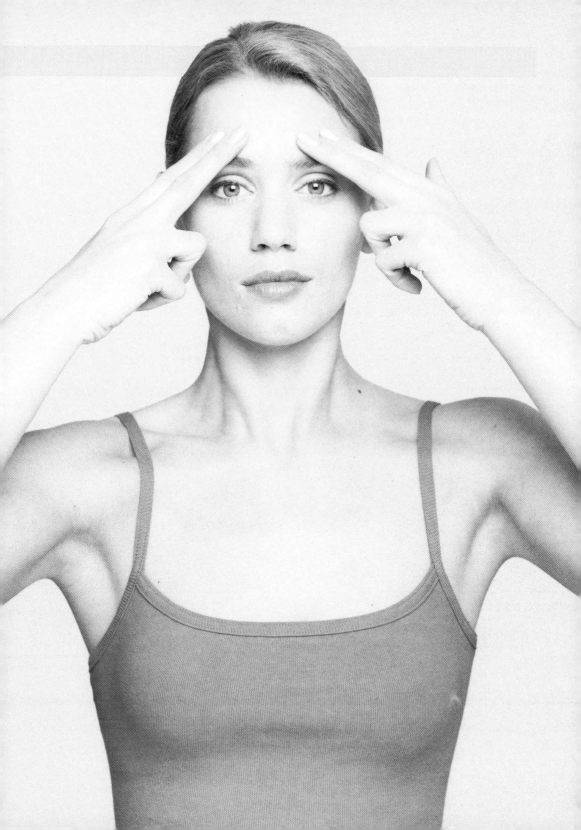

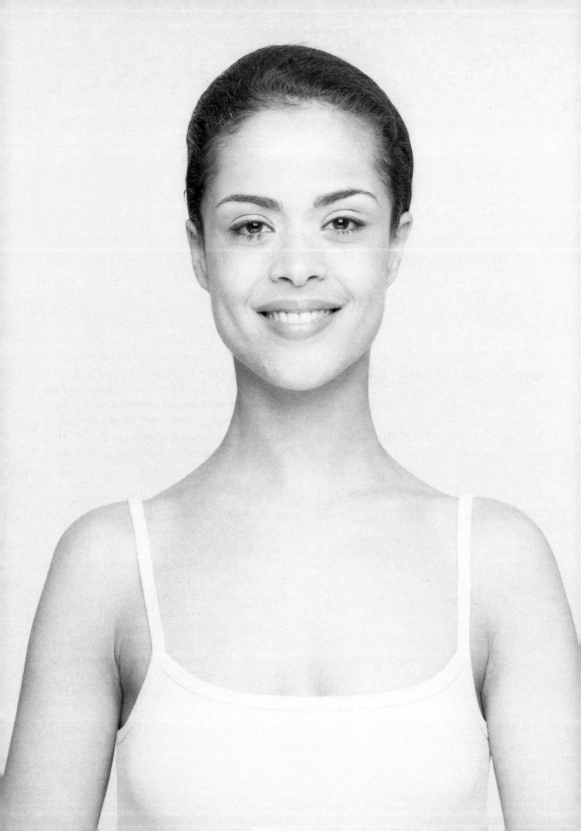

Your Best Asset

 Not everyone likes the telephone. Those who dislike it often say that using it feels incomplete, like half a conversation. Perhaps this is because they are missing the vital visual cues that we take for granted in face-to-face conversations.

Without these cues, and relying purely on someone's tone of voice, subtleties of meaning can be very hard to pick up.

Basic facial expressions are pretty much the same the world over. An ecstatic Egyptian is as easy to spot as a delirious Dane; an angry Australian is as hard to miss as a volcanic Venezuelan. But our face is not just limited to expressing basic human emotions such as joy, anger, surprise and sadness, it can communicate dozens of shades of meaning in-between, everything from mild surprise to complete amazement.

The expressions on our face are clear enough to see, but what creates them is often a mystery to many of us. In the following pages we will explore some of the major facial muscles lying just beneath the skin, working continually to create a symphony of expressions, ebbing and flowing with our moods. We will also discover how single muscles work in harmony to create basic expressions.

Understanding how muscles work individually and in groups will help you to get the most out of later exercises and to turn what is a great asset into your best asset.

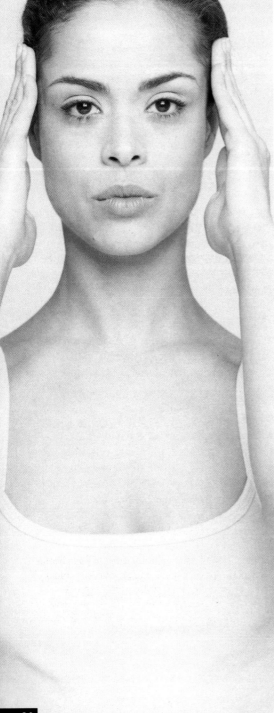

To find the greatest number and variety of muscles in the human body, you need go no further than the face. Nestling closely together, and often over-lapping for compactness and efficiency within a relatively small area, are dozens of agile and powerful muscles of differ-ent shapes and sizes. These muscles are on constant call to perform as we watch, listen to and interact with the world around us.

We begin our exploration of the facial landscape by looking at some key muscles in the fore-head, temples, eyebrows and around the eyes.

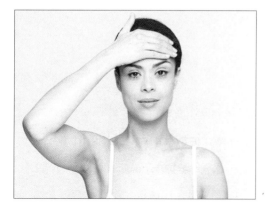

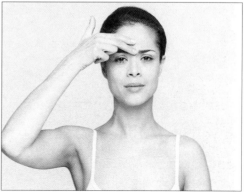

1 Place one hand flat against your forehead and then screw up your forehead. You should feel your hand being pulled up as the large *frontalis* muscle underneath it contracts.

2 Place two fingers in between your eyebrows and frown as if you were disapproving of something. What you are feeling is a combination of the *procerus* and *corrugator supercili* muscles located next to the eyebrows.

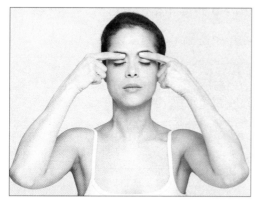

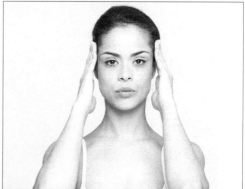

3 Close your eyes and gently place an index finger across the top of each eyelid. Then, keeping your eyes shut, try to lift the eyelid. The thin, delicate muscle you can feel pulling is part of the *orbicularis oculi* encircling the eye.

4 Place your fingers on both sides of your head, slightly above and in front of your ears. Now clench your teeth and feel the wide *temporalis* muscle ripple under your fingers. This muscle is responsible for closing your jaw and helping you to chew.

*Y*ou have to be pretty smart to make it as a facial muscle these days. Not only do you have to be able to handle simple routine tasks such as blinking automatically to cleanse and protect the eyes, but very often you have to track and simultaneously respond to what is happening elsewhere in the face.

To get a good idea of how flexible and well co-ordinated these muscles are, try talking, smiling and eating simultaneously and then for good measure throw in a surprised expression. Confused? Just think what it would be like if you had to consciously plan these moves all the time.

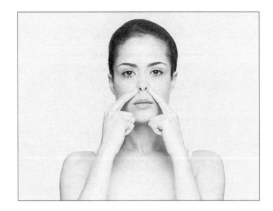

1 Place two fingers on either side of the bridge of the nose to feel the action of the muscles here. Try closing your nostrils with the *compressor naris*, and then – as though you are really angry – flaring your nostrils with *depressor septi*.

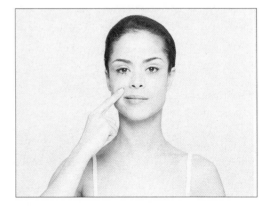

4 Place one finger slightly away from the corner of one side of your mouth and smile to one side. You should be able to feel the *zygomaticus major* muscle contracting under your finger.

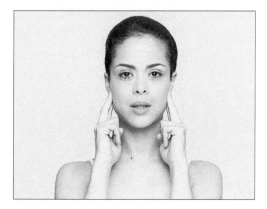

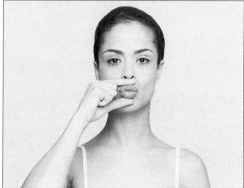

2 Place your fingers on either side of your wisdom teeth and then let your jaw slowly open. You should feel a muscle bulge outwards as you do so. This is the *masseter,* which is a key muscle involved in chewing.

3 Try pursing your lips and feel with your fingers the circular muscle called *orbicularis oris* that surrounds the mouth, without which speaking and kissing would not be quite the same.

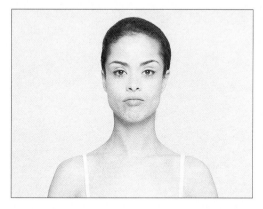

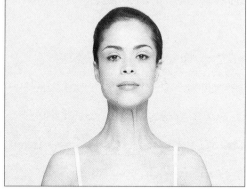

5 This is the muscle that everyone uses when they want to sulk, pout or are about to burst into tears. Simply pull up the muscle at the front of your chin, the *mentalis*.

6 Tense the whole of your neck as if you are just about to explode. A sheath-like muscle, the *platysma,* will stand out and temporarily give you the appearance of a bodybuilder.

𝒲e've already explored some basic individual muscles, so let's now see how they work in tandem by running through some basic facial expressions. It's a good idea to use a mirror to help you see how different muscles work together, but while you practise try to also become aware of how they feel as they flow from one expression to another.

If you do this exercise often enough, your muscles will begin to remember other possibilities. You might notice a sparkle return to your face as you shake off your habitual and perhaps tired facial expression and allow a freshness and vitality to flood in. So go ahead – express yourself.

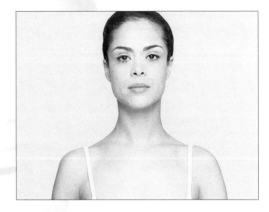

| Start by creating a neutral expression – a fresh canvas, if you like. Breathe slowly, relax your facial muscles and clear your mind so that you can create the following faces.

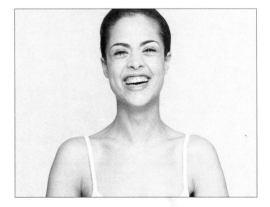

4 Everything has a beginning, middle and end and joy often follows sadness. Think of a really joyful moment in your life and let your face radiate the pure joy of that experience.

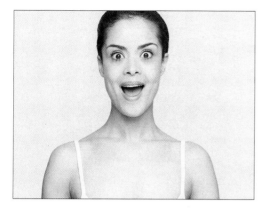

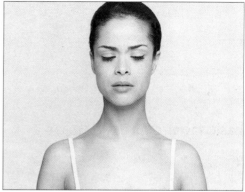

2 Someone has bought you a wonderful, unexpected gift or perhaps you've heard some fantastic news. Let your face show how surprised you are.

3 Sometimes the news we get isn't so great, or things don't turn out quite as we'd hoped. Let your face flow into general disappointment or sadness.

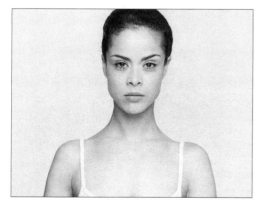

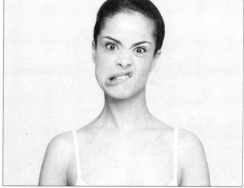

5 OK. So maybe people aren't perfect all the time. What's the one thing that other people do that always makes you really angry? That's right. Show your mirror what you really feel.

6 People who laugh enjoy life more, and if you can't laugh at yourself, this one is definitely for you. Do what you have to, but get silly in front of the mirror. Afterwards return to Step 1.

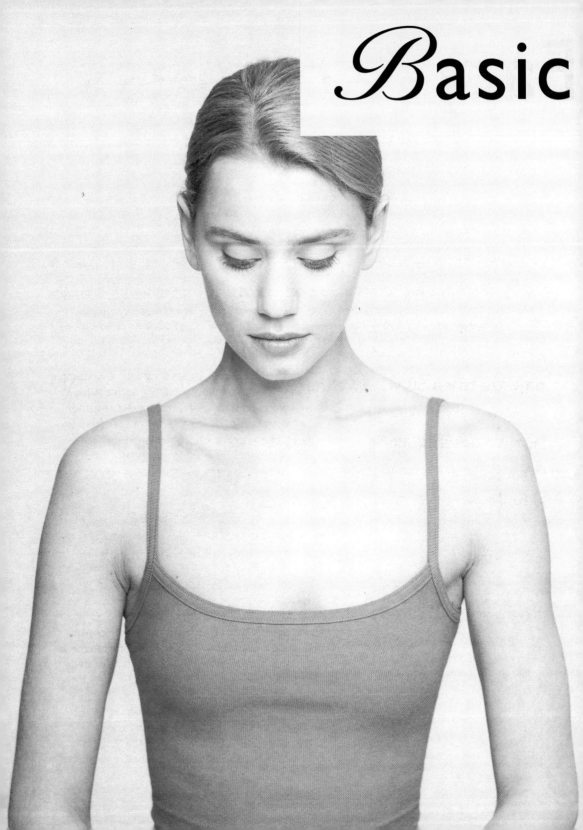

Basic

Facial Fitness

$\mathcal{G}$eorge Orwell once remarked that by the time we reach 50 we have the face we deserve. Poor George, if only he'd regularly practised a basic facial fitness programme!

Fifty years ago skin care regimes and methods of keeping young were in their infancy. Today we have many wonderful techniques for making sure that our skin remains in optimum condition throughout the years and that our faces are as toned as the rest of our bodies.

The basic facial fitness programme is a simple system of exercises, starting with a general warm up, tension-releasing exercises, and then moving on to a series of specific exercises targeting each area within the face, systematically working each major facial muscle, before concluding with an invigorating facial re-energizer.

Some of these exercises may take a little time to get used to and the results may not show immediately, but facial muscles are very responsive and with regular practice your face will start to benefit, giving a more healthy appearance and a glowing complexion as well as a firmer, fitter and more youthful look. It doesn't matter how old you are when you start: the big advantage of this programme is that anyone can benefit at any time of their lives. The important point is that the sooner you start, the sooner you will notice the wonderful benefits the programme has to offer. Practise these basic facial fitness exercises consistently and the vibrant and fresh face you deserve will be yours.

WARMING UP

The first step in any physical programme is warming-up. Although the basic facial programme is a gentle programme, we can benefit from loosening the upper body, specifically the neck and shoulders, which stimulates the circulation, to prepare us for what is to follow and make the facial exercises more effective long-term.

Choose a comfortable chair that also gives you support as you carry out these exercises and the ones that follow. Ensure too that the surrounding environment is well-heated, because muscles relax and function better when they are warm. Finally, make sure that you are wearing loose, comfortable clothing that allows you to move freely as you work through the programme.

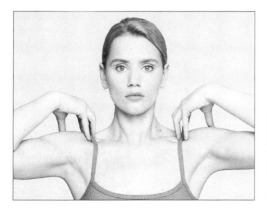 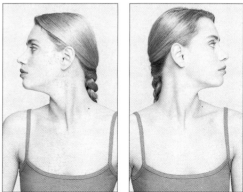

1 Start your warm-up by loosening your shoulders. Place one hand on each shoulder and start to draw clockwise circles with your elbows. Draw these circles progressively larger.

2 Then, keeping your head vertical, slowly look across to your left shoulder and then over to your right. Repeat ten times.

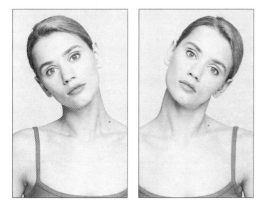 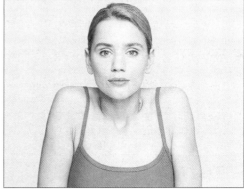

3 Bring your head back to the centre and then gently tilt your head slightly to the left. Bring back to the centre and then repeat on the other side. Continue until you reach a tilt of 45°.

4 Finally, raise your shoulders up to your ears and then allow them to drop down again. Repeat this invigorating movement ten times and end by shaking out.

RELAXING THE FACE

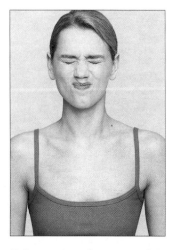

How tense is your face? My bet is that like most people, myself included, your facial muscles are surprisingly tense and longing for some TLC.

I Squeeze your face up as tightly as you can and then let it all go. Repeat ten times.

One of the surest ways of ageing faster than we should is to ignore the tension that builds up in the facial muscles as a result of everyday living. Tension creates blockage and pollution in muscles which can cause more and more lines and wrinkles to form as the surrounding tissues become increasingly stagnant and lifeless. Relax your face, enjoy the surge of energy and feeling of vitality and the rest will follow naturally.

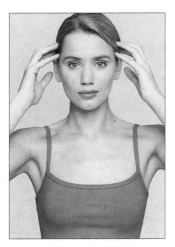

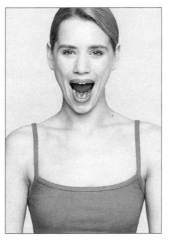

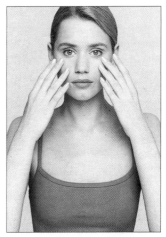

2 Place your hands on either side of your skull, just above your ears and use all your fingers to work the *temporalis* muscles.

3 Now look straight ahead. Let your jaw drop as wide as you can, breathe slowly and create the biggest smile you can. Hold for as long as possible. Relax and repeat ten times. This exercise releases tension from deep within your face.

4 Finally, use your fingertips to explore your face, searching for any remaining tension spots that need to be soothed away. End by gently resting both hands over your face.

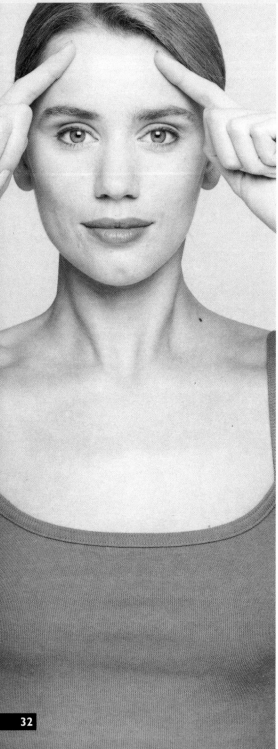

*T*he appearance of worry lines on the forehead is not usually a happy occasion because it marks our eligibility for promotion as one of life's veterans. While some people look forward to promotion, others would prefer to choose when they would like to accept the post. If you feel that promotion has come a little too soon for your liking or you want to put if off as long as possible, then use the following techniques. These can help to banish unwanted worry lines while encouraging extra blood flow and vitality to the whole of the face. So without further ado, let's take it from the top.

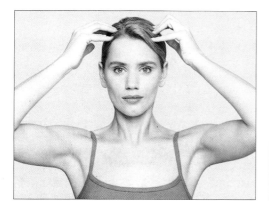

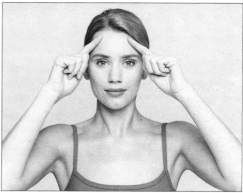

I Place the pads of your fingers firmly on your scalp and massage in small circles, releasing any tension wherever you find it. Tension within the scalp is a great cause of worry lines.

2 Place your index fingers flat against the centre of your forehead. Begin a gentle sawing action up and down, working slowly out and then back in again. Repeat ten times.

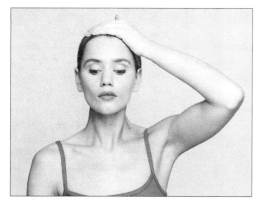

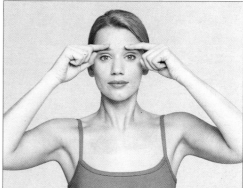

3 Place your hand against the top of your hair-line and look down. This should create a strong stretch that helps to reduce wrinkles and tone the muscle. Relax and repeat ten times.

4 Place your index fingers over your eyebrows and try to contract the *frontalis* muscle while keeping the fingers firmly against the brows. Relax and repeat ten times.

The eyes are the focal point of the face. Stress and tiredness can soon take their toll and leave the thin, delicate skin of this area vulnerable to the first signs of ageing. In use all day, and even pressed into service while we dream at night, our eyes need to be regularly looked after. Use these exercises to keep the eyes and surrounding areas well toned to avoid those first tell-tale signs of advancing years, such as drooping eyelids and crow's feet.

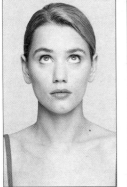 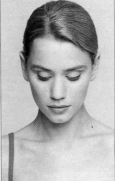 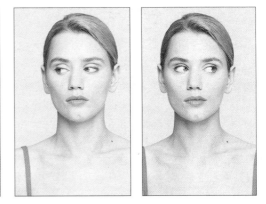

This ancient yoga exercise is excellent for stimulating and relaxing the set of muscles that control eye movement.

Slowly look straight up and down. Next look out of the corner of your eyes, first to the left and then to the right.

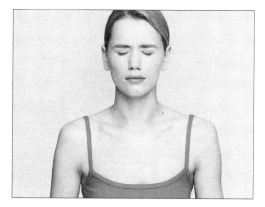

2 Screw up your eyes tightly. Hold for five seconds and release. Repeat ten times.

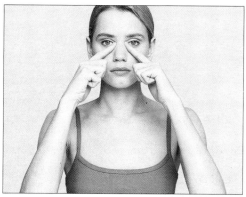

3 With your index fingers, press on the inner corners of both eyes. This is a powerful acupressure point which disperses tension and is good for bags under the eyes.

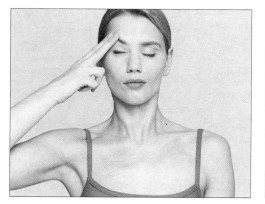

4 Place the index and middle fingers by the outer edge of one eyebrow. While pushing up towards the hairline, look at the tip of your nose, then shut your eye. Relax and repeat ten times before repeating on the other side. This tones the *orbicularis oculi* and is good for droopy eyelids.

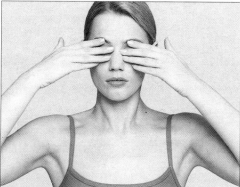

5 Most importantly, rest the eyes. Simply close both eyes and place the palms of your hands over them for as long as you like. You will find the darkness and warmth of your hands produces a rare and delicious sensation.

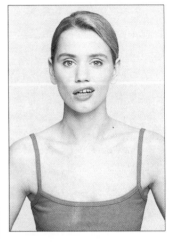

Open your lips slightly and then slowly raise one side of your mouth upwards in a snarl. Hold for a few moments and then release and repeat on the other side. Repeat five times on each side.

$\mathscr{P}$lump, rosy cheeks are a sign of a healthy appearance. However, gravity can begin to make its presence felt as the years roll by, with our cheeks slowly beginning to lose their fullness and starting to sag. The following exercises are designed to reverse this process by stimulating and toning the muscles that support the cheeks. Practise this regularly and you will soon begin to experience the full benefits of keeping gravity in check with stronger and more youthful-looking cheeks.

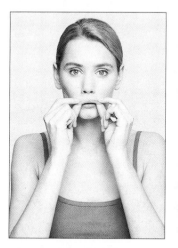

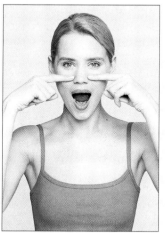

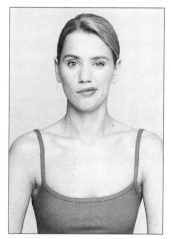

2 Grasp your upper lip and pull down slightly. Now apply the snarl movement, slowly lifting both sides of your mouth. Keep your hold on the lip and feel the cheek muscles being worked.

3 Place your index fingers at the top of each cheek. Open your mouth and slowly move the upper and lower lips away from each other, forming an oval. Smile and feel the cheek muscles being worked under your fingers. Repeat ten times.

4 Now, try to wink one eye without actually closing it. You should feel the cheek muscles rising as you do so. Repeat several times before doing the same exercise with the other cheek.

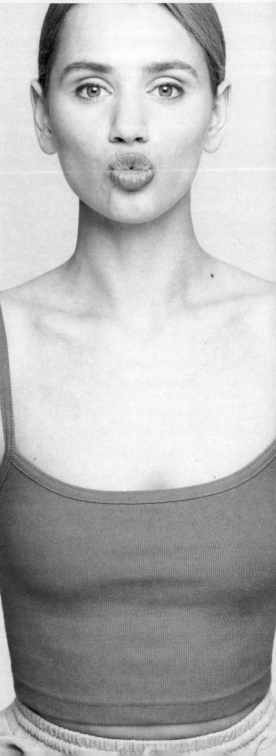

The mouth is one of the hardest-working parts of the human body, with eleven muscles helping us to shape our vowels and words, giving form to our ideas. We also depend on the flexibility of our mouth to highlight what we feel — smiling, laughing, even kissing would be very different if we couldn't use the muscles around our mouth. At the same time, our mouth is at the frontline of the digestive process, keeping food in while we chew it well. If you want your mouth to retain its flexibility and look good through the years, try these exercises to stimulate and tone it.

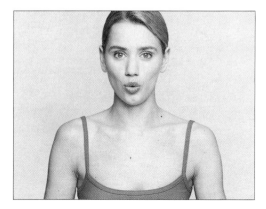

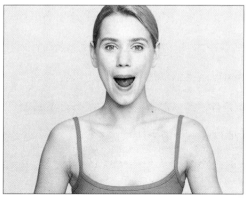

1 Some vowel exercises to start! Say 'A' loudly, shaping it clearly with your lips. Follow with the big vowels: 'E', 'U' and 'O'.

2 Open your mouth halfway, curl your lips inwards. Tense and hold for a few seconds, relax and repeat five times.

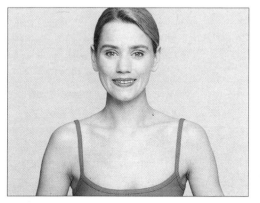

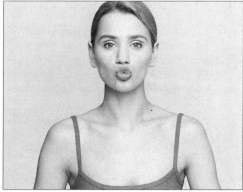

3 Stretch both sides of your mouth outwards, as though you were saying 'Eeee'. Hold for a few moments, relax slowly and repeat five times.

4 Now for the big moment! Pucker your lips for the world's biggest kiss and let fly. Repeat five times or more.

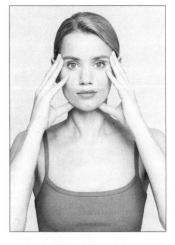

| Place your fingers on either side of the jaw and hook your thumbs just underneath it, by the ears. Let your thumbs slowly sink in, feel the tissue soften, release your thumbs and move along slightly and repeat.

$\mathcal{O}$ne of the most common anxieties about appearance occurs when the jawline suddenly starts to lose its definition and becomes a little vague about where it thinks it is meant to be. If your jawline is beginning to migrate south, don't panic! Left to continue its travels, it might well decide to sign its emigration papers and develop into a double chin, but if you take positive steps now, you will probably be able to convince it to stay put.

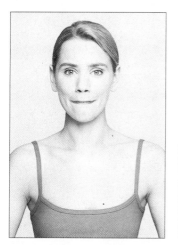

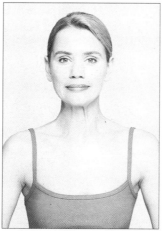

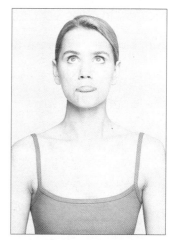

2 Curl your lips over the upper and lower teeth and close your mouth gently. See if you can make a seal-like puckering noise by opening your mouth slightly and sucking in some air briefly before closing.

3 Take a slow, deep breath. Then contract the *platysma* muscle in your neck for three seconds. Relax and repeat ten times.

4 Gently tilt your head back and let your mouth fall slightly open. Keeping your head in this position, bring your lower lip up to meet the upper lip. This move will tone both your neck and jaw.

RE-ENERGIZING THE FACE

After doing the exercises in the basic facial programme, you'd expect to look like you've always lived on a health farm on top of a mountain. But you don't just want muscles that have been toned and stimulated, you also want a full recharge! This is where the exercises below will come in useful. So let's re-energize and go for the tingle!

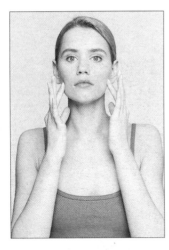

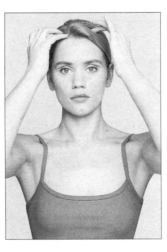

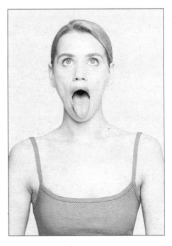

1 Use the pads of your fingers to gently drum all over your face. Start at the chin and work your way up and come down again. Keep going until you can feel your face starting to tingle.

2 Continue up onto your scalp and keep drumming all over your head. This feels great and is wonderful for releasing stored energy in your body.

3 Breathe out through your mouth, stretch your tongue out and down, roll your eyeballs upwards and roar loudly like a lion. This ancient yoga exercise is a powerful toner for your entire face.

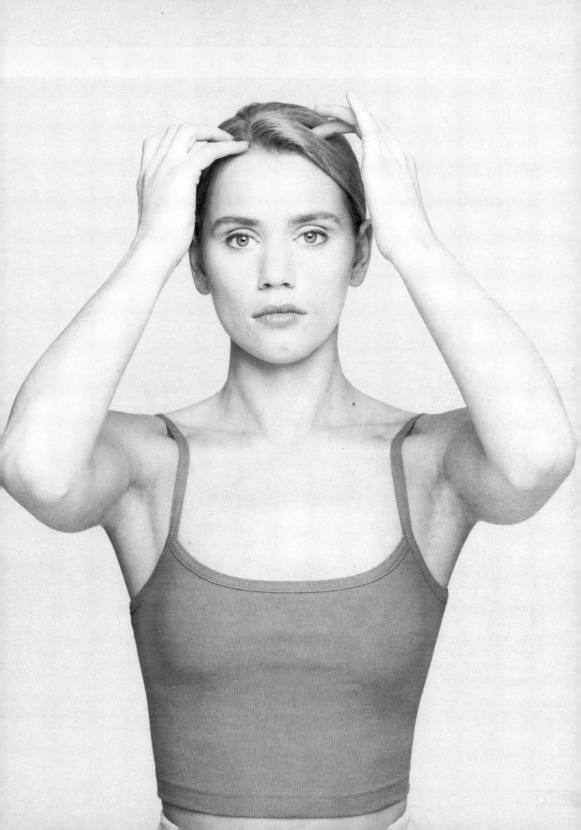

Turning

Back The Clock

 The basic facial fitness programme is a great way to make the most of your face, ensuring that your muscles receive regular attention and remain well toned and healthy.

Unfortunately, not all areas of the face are equal: some need a little extra help now and again in order to firm up in line with the rest of the face. Perhaps your own cheeks are full and rosy, but you'd really like to do something with that second chin. Or maybe you don't mind the odd line here and there, but you really want to pack those bags under the eyes and send them as far away as possible.

This section includes specific exercises to tackle the major problems that the face experiences as it ages. These include: pale skin, loose flesh, wrinkles and expression lines, low eyebrows, crow's feet, bags under the eyes, a downturned mouth, poor jaw definition, a double chin and a lined or 'crêpey' neck.

Some of the exercises, especially those involving the connective tissue in the face, can bring noticeable results if they are practised regularly and with sensitivity, helping you gently to turn back the clock. If any of the above problems are of concern to you, include the specified exercises in your general basic routine. Alternatively, this section can serve as an advanced workout, allowing you to systematically work through the exercises as part of a preventative programme and encouraging your face to look its very best for as long as possible.

PALE SKIN

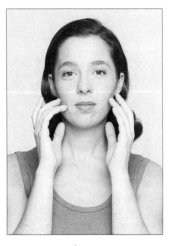

Begin by using the pads of your fngers to tap your face. Make sure you tap the whole face several times.

$\mathscr{O}$ur skin type can change greatly as we get older. With the arrival of the menopause, changes in the circulation within the face can also occur, making us look drawn and as if we spend a lot of time indoors.

Like any other part of the body, the muscles in the face need to be well supplied with blood. This not only brings fresh oxygen and nutrients, but can also take away toxins so that the tissues remain vibrant and healthy. By following these simple exercises, we can keep the energy flowing throughout our face and restore the colour to our cheeks.

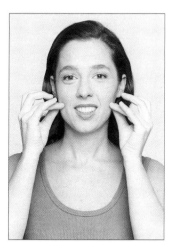 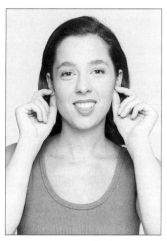 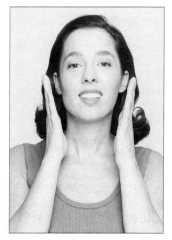

2 Use the fourth fingers of both hands to gently pinch or pluck your cheeks and surrounding the areas.

3 Move onto your ears and give them a thorough massage with your fingers.

4 Finally, gently slap your face with the inside of your hand, pushing the flesh slightly upwards as you do.

LOOSE FLESH

The physical effects of gravity begin to make themselves more apparent as the years go by. This is especially true for the face, where previously well-defined features cast off their anchors and one-by-one set sail due south.

In addition to regularly using the basic programme to benefit your whole face, it's worth trouble-shooting and toning any areas that you think might need extra help. If you practice these exercises regularly, you should see the muscles slowly toning up and become firmer and more defined.

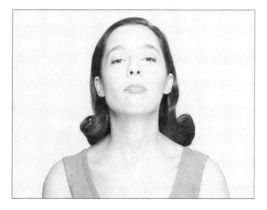

1 Tilt your head back, push out your chin slightly and bring your lower lip over the upper lip.

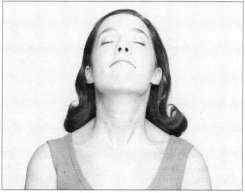

2 Slowly smile in an upwards and outwards direction. Repeat five times.

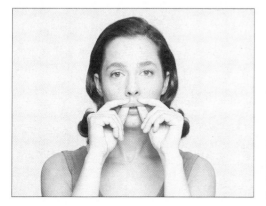

3 Grasp the upper lip and gradually lift the cheek muscles in the direction of the eyes, then release. Repeat five times.

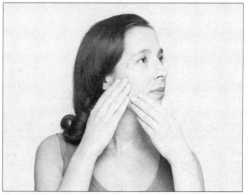

4 To end, use the pads of your fingers to gently caress your face in an upwards direction.

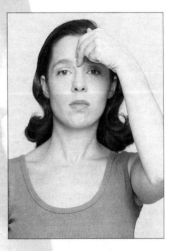

*W*rinkles and expression lines rarely get good press. Consequently, as soon as they appear, they are often resented and wished far away. In truth, they are a natural by-product of life itself, a physical diary of our experiences through the years, signs of who we really are.

▌ Use two fingers to press gently between the eyebrows. This powerful pressure point helps to release deep facial tension.

However, if you'd rather live without them, try the following exercises. As you work, wait patiently for the tissues between your fingers to soften or warm up, because this shows that wrinkle-causing blockages or tensions are being released. Through time, practice and repetition, the lines will slowly become less etched and noticeable, and the skin smoother.

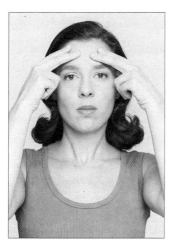 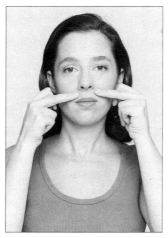 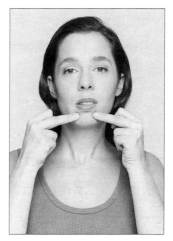

2 Place two fingers slightly apart on the forehead, and bring them slowly closer as you feel the space in between warm up and soften.

3 Use the same technique on the upper lip, slowly working your way around the mouth, releasing tension as you go.

4 Continue in the chin area, working in as many places as you can.

LOW EYEBROWS

$\mathscr{S}$ooner or later, low eyebrows or drooping eyelids will appear in most people's lives. Gravity and the relative thinness of a few muscles that can easily lose their tone through the years are largely to blame for this. Sagging in this area can be particularly worrisome because the face depends on the eye region to help lend it definition. If the shape or size of our eyes is affected, and especially if they are made to appear smaller, the face can 'age'. The way to help prevent this is to exercise the eyebrows and upper eyelids regularly, as shown.

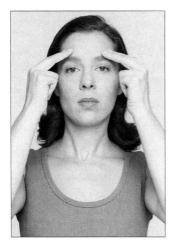

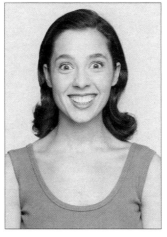

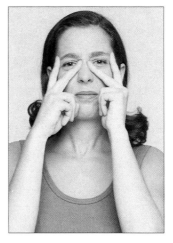

1 With your fingertips, tap backwards and forwards along the eyebrow several times to release tension.

2 Raise your eyebrows as high as you can. Try to do this in four stages. Stretch your eyes as wide open as you can and then bring your eyebrows down slowly, look downwards and then relax. Repeat five times.

3 Create a 'V' shape with your first two fingers and place them on either side of the eyebrows. Now try to squint with both eyes while using your fingers to resist the movement. This is very good for building up the muscles here.

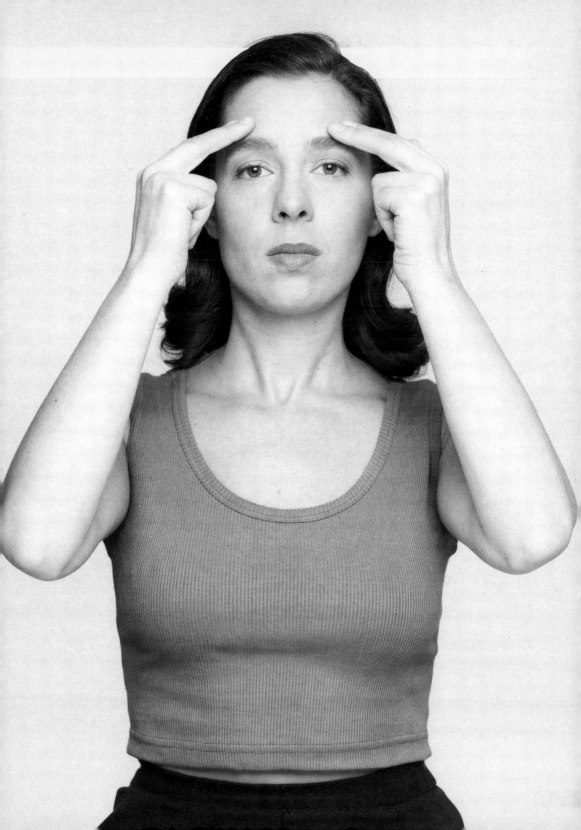

One of the first tell-tale signs that we are getting older is the appearance of lines around our eyes. Many people are sent into a tailspin by this, checking obsessively for new lines every time they pass a mirror. Bags or puffiness in the eye area, which can make us look somewhat tired and world-weary, has a similar effect. If you want to reverse this process, try the exercises below. These will help to release the congestion that creates new lines and deepens existing ones.

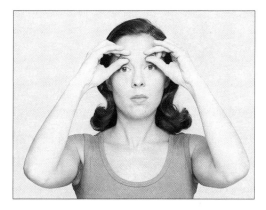

1 Grasp the skin on either side of your eyebrows and roll it between your fingertips. This breaks up a lot of the tension that causes crow's feet.

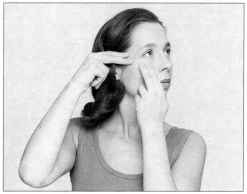

2 Place two fingers on either side of a wrinkle you want to smooth out. Wait for the area between your fingers to warm up and soften, letting the crow fly away!

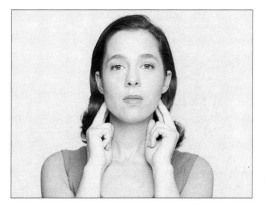

3 Use two fingers to massage free any congestion that has built up immediately behind the earlobe. Congestion in this area can contribute to bags forming under the eyes.

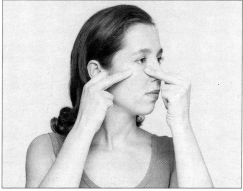

4 Use the same technique as in Step 2 to soften and release congestion below the eye. The skin here is delicate, so be very gentle as you work.

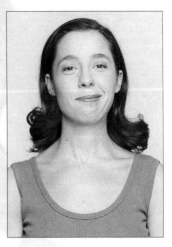

*A*fter many years the smiling muscles on either side of the mouth (*zygomaticus major* and *minor*) can start to lose their tone, causing the corners of the mouth to turn downwards, creating an appearance of sulking or frowning. No one wants to look perpetually frumpy, so the answer is to make sure that these muscles are regularly exercised properly to restore tone and lift the corners so that the mouth is level once again.

I With your mouth slightly open, bring the corners of the left side of your mouth out as far as possible. Then work the right-hand side of your mouth. Repeat five times.

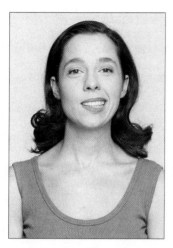

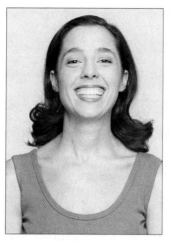

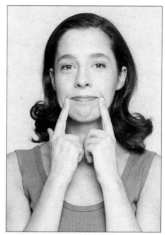

2 Close your lips and with one side of your mouth, smile broadly up towards the ears. Work the other side and repeat. Once you can do this successfully, try both sides at the same time.

3 Repeat Step 2, but this time extend the smile up towards your eyes. When you are ready, work both sides simultaneously.

4 Finally, place your index fingers on the corners of your mouth and tense the corners into an upward smile. Use your fingers as resistance and then relax. Repeat twenty times.

DOUBLE TROUBLE

These two exercises are designed to help you keep a well-defined jawline. This is essential if you don't want little folds of flesh to appear and give your face a loose, even droopy appearance. If the muscles underneath the chin also begin to lose their tone and fall under gravity's spell, then they too can begin to sag, encouraging the development of a double chin, which can look less than flattering. If you practise these techniques regularly, you can help chase away the spectre of loose folds and unwanted chins, creating well-toned muscles and smoother, tauter skin.

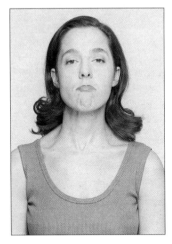 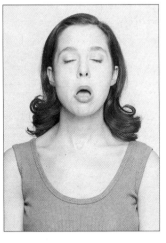 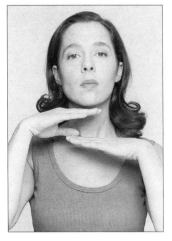

1 Open your mouth and pull your lower lip tightly over the bottom teeth.

Then open and close your jaw as if you were trying to scoop something up with it. Make sure you really work your jaw so that you tone the muscles. Repeat five times.

2 This is a classic move for toning slack muscles. Use the back of your hand to tap or gently slap under your chin. Repeat with the other hand and increase your speed.

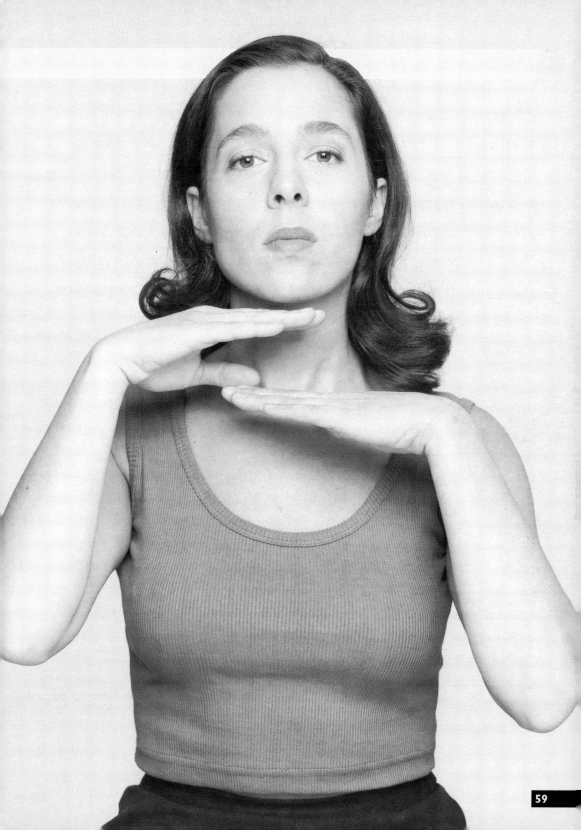

$\mathscr{T}$here are some lucky individuals who weather the passing years with hardly a line or fold; the only place that gives away their age is their neck. The skin in this area is very thin and its natural elasticity and smoothness can slowly change, drying and becoming crêpe-like as we get older. In addition, lines can easily appear on the neck itself, slowly deepening into creases. If you want to preserve the smooth quality of your neck or return it to its former glory, then spend some time investing in these exercises.

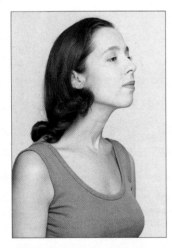

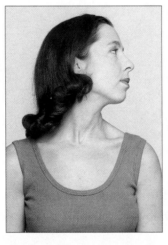

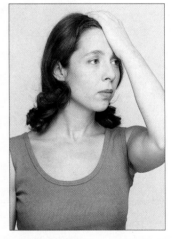

1 Tense your neck muscles and stick your neck out slowly and bring it right back like a turtle. Repeat five times.

2 Keeping your muscles tense, turn your head from side to side five times. This is excellent for toning the neck muscles, preventing slackness.

3 Place your hand on your forehead and push forward with your head, resisting with your hand. Repeat by putting the hand on the back of the head and pushing backwards.

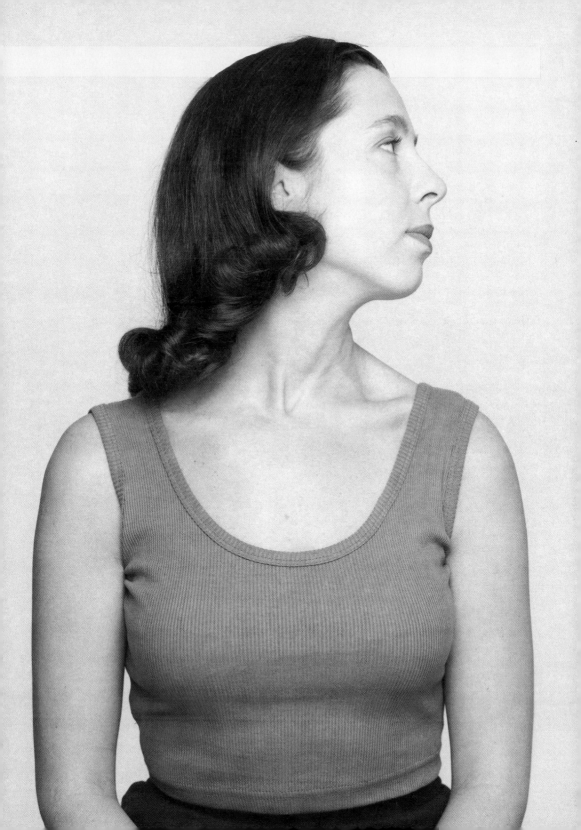

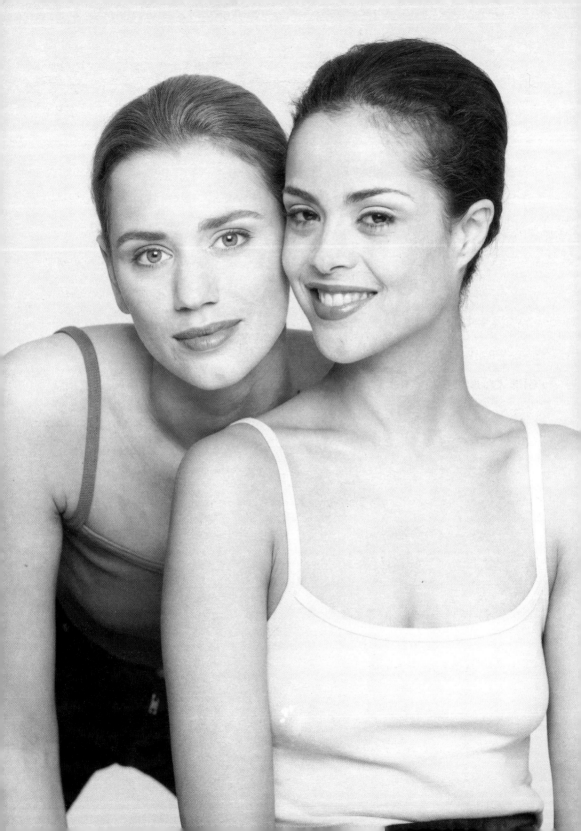

Facial Harmony

 If you feel that your facial muscles are over-worked, tired and truly in need of a holiday away from it all, then pamper yourself and get your partner to give you one of the following fabulous facial massages.

While it is important to make sure that you follow and practise the basic facial fitness programme and regularly target any specific areas that need special attention, it's also a good idea – if you can find the time – to receive a soothing facial massage.

The results are always quite beautiful to watch: the face slowly relaxes, deep-seated tension is unlocked and caressed away and the years gently rolled back, leaving your face looking softer, fresher and years younger.

Regular massage is an extremely powerful tool because it successfully disperses the tension that builds up in the muscles and tissues, thus preventing the formation of lines and wrinkles. It also helps to restore circulation and clears out any harmful and ageing toxins trapped in the tissues.

In the following pages we will look at two types of massage. The first is a wonderful relaxer and general tension disperser which requires a tiny amount of oil mixed with lavender to work its magic. The second uses no oil at all and releases tension at the deepest level, smoothing out long-term wrinkles. These sequences are suggestions, ideas to be explored, so encourage your partner to develop his or her own intuition and creativity in their search for facial harmony.

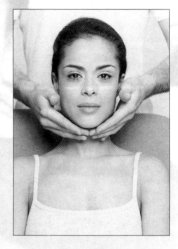

If you've never worked with oil or given a massage before, don't worry. Massage is one of our most ancient skills and once you get started, your fingers will begin to remember and guide you in what to do.

▌ Place your hands on either side of your partner's face at the base of the neck and slowly stroke upwards towards the forehead. Repeat three times.

You'll need some almond, grapeseed or olive oil; sufficient just to fill the bottom of a cup. Mix a couple of drops of lavender, an all-purpose essential oil, and dab just a little of the mixture on your hands to rub into the palms. Make sure your hands are warm before slowly bringing them towards your partner to start.

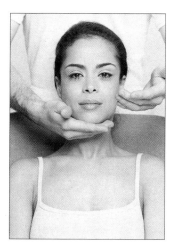

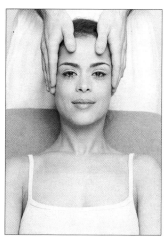

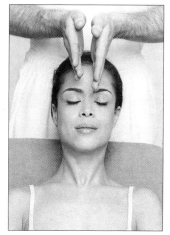

2 Gently caress underneath the chin, using alternate hands in upward sweeping movements.

3 Position your thumbs in the middle of the forehead and slowly move your thumbs away from each other to the sides of the head.

4 Using the underside of the little fingers, create a light friction between your partner's eyebrows.

Gently encourage your partner to breathe out all their tension. Once you begin to work, make sure that all your attention is completely on them. Losing physical connection can be very disconcerting for your partner and can stop them from fully relaxing and enjoying the benefits of the massage.

Keep your movements small, the pressure constant and the speed even. Don't rush any movement; if anything, slow down and repeat the same one several times, because this will help your partner to relax deeply and really let go. Focus on releasing any tension and smoothing out any lines you may find: you might be surprised to see real changes happening as you work.

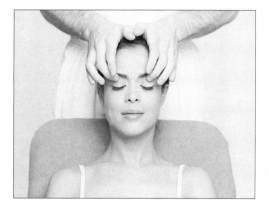

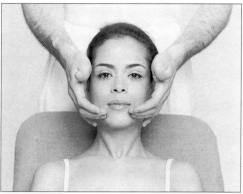

1 Place your third fingers just underneath the brow bone and press upwards and then repeat, moving outward until you reach the outer edge of the eyebrow.

2 Use your fourth fingers to create small upward circles around the chin.

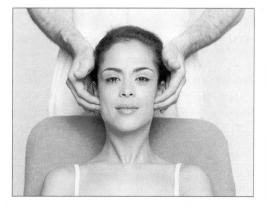

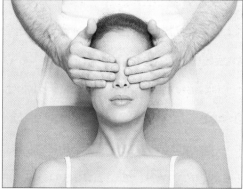

3 Find the chewing muscles on each side of the face. Make some slow circles with the pads of your fingers.

4 Grasp the ears and gently pull outwards. Finish by covering your partner's eyes for a few moments.

*A*lthough oil-based facials are very pleasurable to receive and help release general tension, nothing beats working without oil when you want more detailed, close-up work.

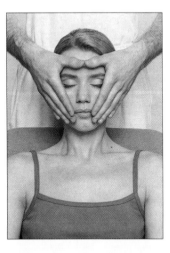

Gently place both hands over your partner's face. This will feel good and is very calming.

The aim when you work is to release tissues, some of which may be trapped together in small pockets. This requires the lightest of pressure upon the skin and the patience to wait for the tissue to slowly release. If you place one or two fingers on either side of such a pocket and wait, you will slowly begin to feel the area warm and soften. When it does so, move your fingers slightly closer together and repeat until the tension has completely disappeared.

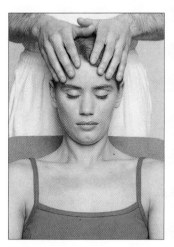 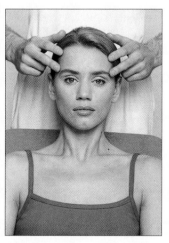 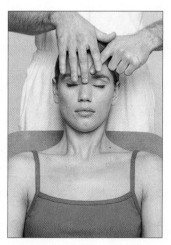

2 Spread your fingers and place them very, very lightly on the forehead, then begin to move towards the hairline, feeling for subtle restrictions.

3 Place your first two fingers on either side of the forehead and wait till you feel a slight warming-up or release. Move the fingers a little closer and repeat.

4 Put one finger on the bridge of the nose and hold it there for support as you run the index finger of the other hand down the nose.

*T*his approach works on the connective tissue, the flesh that is not muscle and which binds everything together: skin, muscle, tendons and organs. When a kink or blockage occurs in this tissue, it can mean the beginning of wrinkles. By working directly on the connective tissue, we can see even quite deep wrinkles fade and disappear.

The other technique to develop when using no oil is to work an area in several directions, repeating the same movement over and over again. Connective tissue has many layers and working like this will guarantee success.

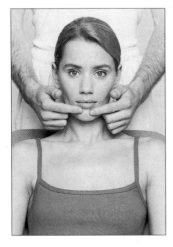 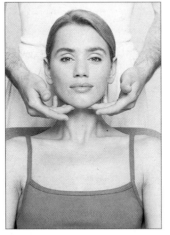 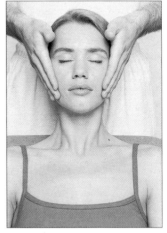

1 Begin by searching for any restrictions on the upper and lower lip. Again, move the fingers closer when an area softens, then repeat.

2 Repeat the process, this time working around the chin. Don't forget to try different directions.

3 Place your fingers under your partner's chin and wait for a warming-up, softening or pulsation in the area between your fingers.

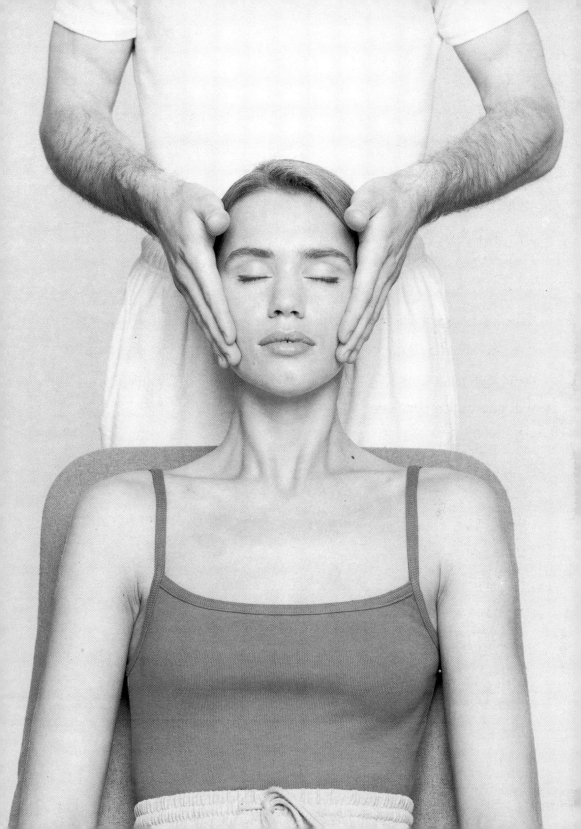

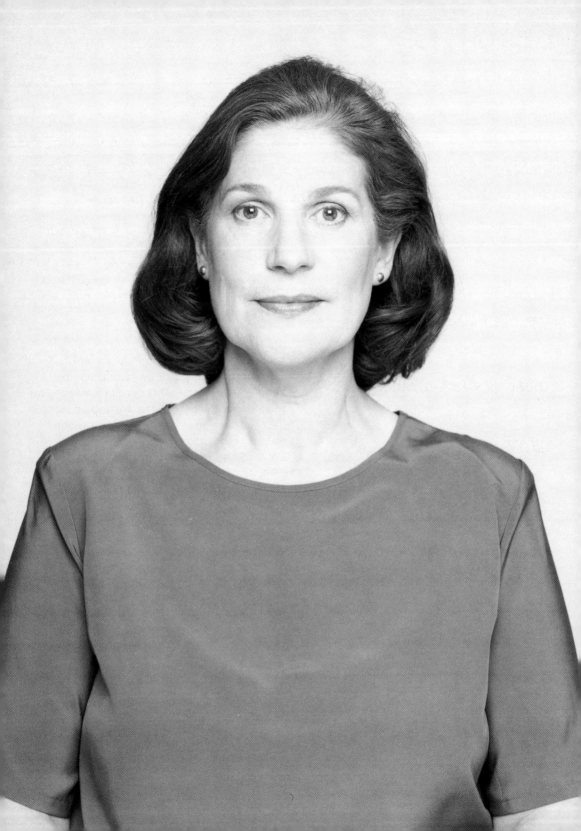

Less Is More

 *L*et's face it, the last thing you want to hear as you get older is how great your make-up looks. Wouldn't you much rather be told how great you look?

But if you want to keep looking your very best throughout the years, it's important that you adapt to change. As you blossom into sophistication and wisdom, you probably won't want to go on wearing the same clothes you did as a teenager. Many women, however, stick to the same make-up ideas first learnt as young girls. Unfortunately, the brash colour schemes that once impressed your friends will probably fail to keep up with the changes in your face or skin tone as you mature. Rather than complimenting you, vibrant colours can often make you look considerably older than you are.

At the first signs of ageing it's easy to fall into the trap of applying more and more make-up in the hope that no one will notice that you're getting older. But it's hard to fool any-one when your make-up enters a room before you do.

It takes only a subtle shift of focus – accentu-ating the positive, enhancing your eyes rather than hiding your crow's feet – to look ten years younger. By updating your techniques and colour schemes, adapting to changes in your face and being subtle in your use of make-up, you can make the most of what nature has given you. Whatever your age, you can look fresh, radiant, attractive and confident. It really is true: less is more.

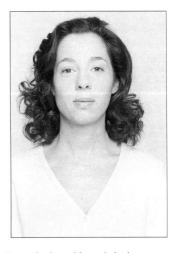

Foundation: Use a light base and cover face and neck. Then gently press in translucent powder to fix your foundation.

*B*eing a 30-something is not easy. It's a time when we get on with the serious business of settling down, developing a career and building a home and family. Any one of these is a full-time job in itself: juggling all three successfully sometimes verges on the impossible.

It's also a time when we start to notice the first subtle signs of ageing, with lines and perhaps a change in our skin appearing. Gone are the days when we could do exactly what we wanted to our body. Now we really need to look after ourselves and learn how to use make-up in a way that naturally enhances our beauty.

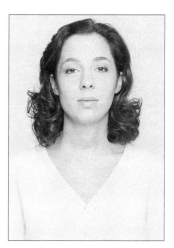 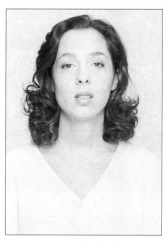 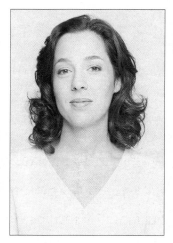

Eyes: Using a cream colour, highlight the lower eyelid and just below the eyebrow. Then use some brown on the crease between the browbone and eyelid to create a contour effect and blend. Apply eyeliner to the upper and lower lid and blend once more.

Lips: Line with a soft pencil and then use a moisturizing lip colour to cover lips.

Colour: Whereas a blusher is used to bring out pale cheeks, a bronzer can be used to bring colour to the whole face. Gently bronze the face and highlight the cheek bones to give a healthy glow.

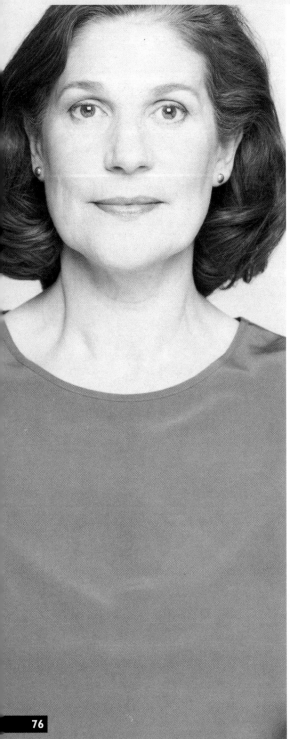

*L*ife does begin at 40, with many women experiencing greater energy and drive. On the other hand, they also have to cope with the great physical upheavals that the menopause brings.

Facial skin often changes, becoming less plump, looser and more lined and skin type can change dramatically. Using the same make-up techniques will only add to the ageing process, so it's important to update and learn how to accept and adapt to the new you. This make-over will show you some ideas, but any cosmetics sales assistant will be more than happy to spend time discussing appropriate colours, techniques and products to suit your personal needs.

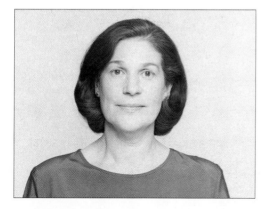

Foundation: If dark bags have settled, you can use a cover-up before you apply your base. Don't go too heavy as this will make the skin appear older. Gently powder with translucent powder.

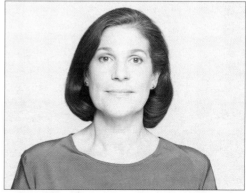

Eyes: Cover the eyelid with a non-metallic cream/white shadow and add contour shadow just above the socket line as described in page 75. Blend. Then pencil the outer third of the eyes lightly and blend using a Q-tip.

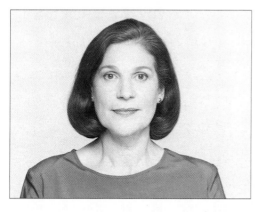

Lips: If you have fine lines around your mouth, use a dry lip liner. Any other type of lip liner may tend to bleed up the lines. Then apply colour. If you want your colour to last, blot with tissue, powder and apply lip colour again.

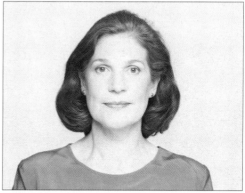

Colour: Just for the final touch, apply a small amount of bronzer all over your face to give a hint of colour.

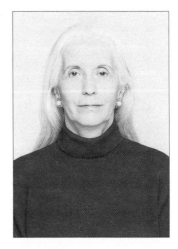

$\mathcal{T}$here are many mature women who could give their younger sisters a run for their money. What they have in common is a graceful acceptance of their age and the determination to use all their resources intelligently to help them look like a million dollars.

They take consistent good care of their skin, recognize and highlight their best features, regularly revise their make-up, and embrace any physical change as an integral part of themselves. And, if their eyesight is less than perfect, a magnifying mirror helps them to put their make-up on accurately and to keep it light, refreshing and natural.

Foundation: On a well moisturized skin gently apply your base, carefully blending the hair line and the jaw and neck. Try not to get any in your hair especially if your hair is light or grey. Then gently powder by pressing with a power puff.

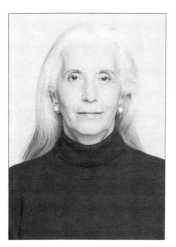

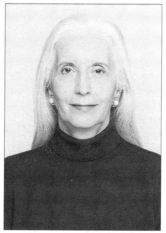

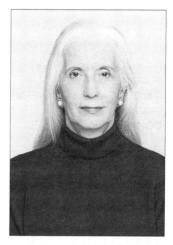

Eyes: Using non-metallic shadow, cover the eye area with a cream right up to the brow. Then lightly blend a brown shadow above the socket line which is where your eyelid dips in. Then blend. Apply eye pencil to the outer third using gentle strokes.

Lips: Apply a tinted lip moisturizer. This is sometimes better than a colour if your lipstick tends to bleed.

Colour: Whereas a blusher is used to bring out pale cheeks, a bronzer can be used to bring colour to the whole face. Apply a bronzer all over your face using a big brush and light strokes to create a healthy glow.

INDEX